CALORIE DEFICIT

COOKBOK

The Ultimate Guide to Quick, Easy and Delicious Low-Calorie Recipe to Lose Weight, Burn Fat and Live a Healthy Lifestyle. Includes a 2 Week Meal Plan

Jolanda David

EMAIL OUTREACH:

Thank you for choosing to embark on this journey with me through the pages of this book. I understand that reading about a subject as personal as diet and nutrition can often raise questions, spark curiosity, which is why I want to offer my assistance to you.

If you find yourself in need of clarification, seeking guidance, or desiring a deeper understanding of the concepts discussed within this book, please feel free to reach out to me via email at: **dietwithjolandadavid@gmail.com** . As a dedicated professional in the field, I am more than happy to provide you with a free consultation to address your queries.

I assure you that I will personally respond within 24 hours, eager to assist you on your path to wellness.

Your feedback and questions are valuable to me, and I am grateful for the opportunity to support you on your journey. Thank you for purchasing this book, and I look forward to connecting with you soon.

TABLE OF CONTENTS

INTRODUCTION

Imagine a world where you can enjoy delicious meals while achieving your weight loss goals. A world where health and flavor collide, and every bite takes you one step closer to your dream body. Welcome to the Calorie Deficit Cookbook, a treasure trove of mouthwatering recipes designed to ignite your taste buds and propel you towards a healthier, happier you.

As a dietitian, I have witnessed countless individuals embark on their weight loss journeys, brimming with determination but often struggling to find the balance between taste and nutrition. It was through one such encounter that I discovered the transformative power of calorie deficit cooking and its ability to revolutionize lives.

Let me introduce you to Amanda, a remarkable woman who entrusted me with her wellness goals. Amanda had battled with weight issues for years, tirelessly seeking a solution that would allow her to shed unwanted pounds without sacrificing the joy of eating. She yearned for a sustainable approach, one that would empower her to make better choices while embracing the flavors she loved.

When Amanda walked into my office that fateful day, her eyes sparkled with both hope and skepticism. She had tried numerous diets and had grown disillusioned with empty promises. But little did she know that her life was about to change forever. I smiled warmly, understanding her reservations but confident in the transformative potential of the calorie deficit approach.

We sat down together, discussing her goals, preferences, and struggles. It was clear that Amanda needed a comprehensive solution—one that combined practicality, nourishment, and culinary delight. And that's when I unveiled the secret weapon: the Calorie Deficit Cookbook.

Intrigued, Amanda eagerly flipped through the pages, her eyes widening as she discovered an array of delectable recipes meticulously crafted to fuel her weight loss journey. From vibrant breakfast smoothies to satiating dinners bursting with flavor, every recipe was carefully calibrated to ensure a calorie deficit without compromising taste.

As we delved into the cookbook, Amanda's skepticism slowly dissolved. She realized that her journey towards a healthier lifestyle didn't have to be filled with deprivation or bland, uninspiring meals. The recipes in this book were her passport to a world of culinary exploration, where she could savor every bite while still staying on track.

Over the course of our time together, Amanda and I embarked on a voyage of discovery. We experimented with colorful veggie creations, flavorful lean protein options, and wholesome whole grain goodness. We crafted nutrient-rich soups and stews, satisfying salads, and mouthwatering wraps. The possibilities were endless, and Amanda couldn't contain her excitement as she reveled in each new culinary adventure.

Week by week, the transformation began. Amanda's energy levels surged, her clothes started to loosen, and her confidence blossomed. The combination of a well-structured calorie deficit and the tantalizing recipes in the cookbook had become her secret formula for success. She no longer dreaded mealtimes; instead, she eagerly looked forward to the next enticing dish that awaited her.

As Amanda's story unfolded, I couldn't help but feel a profound sense of fulfillment. Witnessing her reclaim her health and reignite her love for food was a testament to the transformative power of the calorie deficit approach. It was a reminder that weight loss doesn't have to be a grueling, monotonous journey but rather an opportunity to rediscover the joy of nourishing both body and soul.

And now, it is my honor to share this journey with you. In the pages of this book, you will find not only recipes but also a roadmap to your own transformation. This book is a beacon of hope, guiding you towards a future where healthy living and culinary pleasure coexist harmoniously.

So, join me as we explore the vast array of low-calorie, flavor-packed creations that will tantalize your taste buds, fuel your body, and propel you towards the best version of yourself. Together, we will navigate the world of calorie deficit cooking, empowering you to embrace the abundance of delicious, wholesome meals that await you.

Let this book be your companion on this remarkable journey—a journey that will redefine your relationship with food and unlock the door to a vibrant, energized, and fulfilled life. Get ready to embrace the power of flavors, the art of balance, and the joy of reclaiming your health. The path to transformation begins here, and I invite you to take the first step with me.

CHAPTER 1

UNDERSTANDING CALORIE DEFICIT

WHAT IS A CALORIE DEFICIT?

When it comes to weight loss, a calorie deficit is a fundamental concept. It refers to a situation where you intake a lower amount of calories than what your body requires to sustain its existing weight. In other words, it is an energy imbalance where you're burning more calories than you're consuming. By creating a calorie deficit, you prompt your body to tap into its stored energy reserves, leading to weight loss.

WHY IS CALORIE DEFICIT IMPORTANT FOR WEIGHT LOSS?

Weight loss occurs when your body burns more calories than it takes in, and a calorie deficit is essential for achieving this. When you consistently maintain a calorie deficit over time, your body turns to stored fat as a source of energy. This process helps you shed excess weight and reduce body fat.

Calorie deficit is crucial because it addresses the basic principle of thermodynamics: energy balance. By consuming fewer calories than your body needs, you force it to utilize stored energy, resulting in weight loss. Without a calorie deficit, your body has no incentive to tap into its fat stores and lose weight.

HOW TO DETERMINE YOUR CALORIE DEFICIT

To determine your calorie deficit, you need to calculate the number of calories your body requires to maintain its current weight (also known as maintenance calories) and then consume fewer calories than that.

There are various methods to estimate your maintenance calories. One commonly used approach is the Harris-Benedict equation, which calculates your basal metabolic rate (BMR) and then applies an activity factor to estimate your total daily energy expenditure (TDEE). Several online calculators and smartphone apps can help you determine your maintenance calories based on your age, gender, weight, height, and activity level.

Once you know your maintenance calories, you can create a calorie deficit by reducing your daily calorie intake. A general guideline is to aim for a deficit of 500-1000 calories per day, which can lead to a safe and sustainable weight loss of 1-2 pounds (0.5-1 kg) per week.

TIPS FOR MAINTAINING A CALORIE DEFICIT

Maintaining a calorie deficit can be challenging, but with the right strategies, it is achievable. Here are some helpful tips to help you stay on track:

1. **Track your food intake:** Use a food diary or a calorie-tracking app to monitor your calorie intake. This awareness will help you make mindful choices and stay within your calorie limit.
2. **Focus on nutrient-dense foods:** Opt for whole, unprocessed foods that provide essential nutrients while being relatively low in calories. Vegetables, fruits, lean proteins, whole grains, and healthy fats should form the basis of your diet.
3. **Practice portion control:** Be mindful of portion sizes to avoid unintentionally consuming excess calories. Use measuring cups, a food scale, or visual cues to measure appropriate serving sizes.
4. **Incorporate physical activity:** Combine your calorie deficit with regular exercise to enhance weight loss and improve overall health. Engage in both cardiovascular exercises and strength training to maximize calorie burning and preserve muscle mass.
5. **Seek support and accountability:** Joining a weight loss group or enlisting the support of friends and family can help you stay motivated and accountable. Sharing your goals and progress with others can provide valuable encouragement along your journey.

Remember that creating a calorie deficit is a gradual process, and it's important to prioritize sustainable and healthy weight loss. Gradually reducing your calorie intake and making small, sustainable lifestyle changes can lead to long-term success in achieving and maintaining a healthy weight.

CHAPTER 2
UNDERSTANDING MACRONUTRIENTS

CARBOHYDRATES: FRIEND OR FOE?

Carbohydrates are often the subject of debate when it comes to nutrition and weight management. However, they play a crucial role in providing energy to the body. Carbohydrates are the body's primary source of fuel, particularly for the brain and muscles. These can be found in a variety of foods such as grains, fruits, vegetables, and legumes.

Not all carbohydrates are created equal. There are two main types: complex carbohydrates and simple carbohydrates. Complex carbohydrates, such as whole grains, vegetables, and legumes, contain fiber and are digested more slowly, providing a steady release of energy. Simple carbohydrates, found in sugary foods and refined grains, are quickly digested and can cause rapid spikes in blood sugar levels.

For a healthy diet, it is important to focus on consuming complex carbohydrates while limiting simple carbohydrates. Complex carbohydrates provide essential nutrients and fiber, which aids in digestion, regulates blood sugar levels, and promotes a feeling of fullness. Aim for whole grains, fruits, and vegetables as your primary sources of carbohydrates.

PROTEIN: THE BUILDING BLOCK

Protein is a crucial macronutrient that has a significant function in the development and mending of tissues, the production of enzymes and hormones, and the maintenance of a strong immune system. It consists of amino acids, which serve as the fundamental components of protein. While the body can produce certain amino acids, others need to be acquired from the diet.

Protein-rich foods include meat, poultry, fish, eggs, dairy products, legumes, and tofu. It is crucial to incorporate a diverse range of protein sources into your diet to ensure that you acquire all the necessary amino acids. The recommended daily intake of protein varies based on factors such as age, sex, activity level, and overall health. As a general guideline, aim to consume about 0.8 grams of protein per kilogram of body weight.

Protein not only provides essential nutrients but also contributes to satiety. Including protein in your meals and snacks can help control hunger and prevent overeating. Additionally, protein plays a crucial role in preserving lean muscle mass during weight loss, making it an important component of a calorie deficit diet.

FATS: THE GOOD, THE BAD, AND THE UGLY

Fats have long been demonized in the realm of nutrition, but they are an essential macronutrient that serves several important functions in the body. Fats provide energy, help absorb fat-soluble vitamins, protect organs, insulate the body, and assist in hormone production.

Not all fats are created equal. There are healthy fats, such as monounsaturated and polyunsaturated fats found in foods like avocados, nuts, seeds, and fatty fish. These fats have been linked to various health benefits, including improved heart health and reduced inflammation.

On the other hand, saturated fats and trans fats should be limited in the diet. Saturated fats are found in animal products and high-fat dairy, while trans fats are primarily found in processed and fried foods. These fats have been associated with an increased risk of heart disease and should be consumed sparingly.

When incorporating fats into your diet, focus on the healthy fats while minimizing the intake of saturated and trans fats. It's important to keep portion sizes in mind, as fats are calorie-dense. Aim for a balanced approach, where fats make up a moderate portion of your total calorie intake.

BALANCING MACROS FOR OPTIMAL HEALTH

Achieving a healthy balance of macronutrients is essential for optimal health. Each macronutrient serves a specific purpose and finding the right balance can help support overall well-being.

Aim to include a variety of foods in your diet that provide carbohydrates, protein, and healthy fats. Fill your plate with whole grains, fruits, and vegetables for carbohydrates, lean proteins such as chicken, fish, and legumes, and sources of healthy fats like avocados, nuts, and seeds.

CHAPTER 3

BREAKFAST DELIGHTS

ENERGIZING SMOOTHIES AND SHAKES

1. Green Tea Berry Smoothie

Cook time: 5 minutes

Servings: 2

Ingredients:

- 1 cup brewed green tea, chilled
- 1 cup frozen mixed berries (strawberries, blueberries, raspberries)
- 1 small ripe banana
- 1/2 cup plain Greek yogurt
- 1 tablespoon honey or a natural sweetener (optional)
- Ice cubes (optional)

Instructions:

1. In a blender, combine the chilled green tea, frozen mixed berries, ripe banana, Greek yogurt, and honey (if desired).
2. Blend on high until smooth and well combined.
3. If desired, add a few ice cubes and blend again until the smoothie reaches your desired consistency.
4. Pour into glasses and serve immediately.

Nutritional Information per serving:

Calories: 90 Protein: 5g Carbohydrates: 18g Fat: 0g Fiber: 4g

2. Pineapple Coconut Smoothie

Cook time: 5 minutes

Servings: 2

Ingredients:

- 1 cup unsweetened coconut water
- 1 cup frozen pineapple chunks
- 1 small ripe banana
- 1/4 cup unsweetened coconut flakes
- 1 tablespoon fresh lime juice

Instructions:

1. In a blender, combine the coconut water, frozen pineapple chunks, ripe banana, coconut flakes, and lime juice.
2. Blend on high until smooth and well combined.
3. Pour into glasses and serve immediately.

Nutritional Information per serving:

Calories: 110 Protein: 1g Carbohydrates: 26g Fat: 2g Fiber: 4g

3. Chocolate Almond Protein Shake

Cook time: 5 minutes

Servings: 1

Ingredients:

- 1 cup unsweetened almond milk
- 1 tablespoon unsweetened cocoa powder
- 1 scoop chocolate protein powder
- 1 tablespoon almond butter
- Ice cubes (optional)

Instructions:

1. In a blender, combine the almond milk, cocoa powder, chocolate protein powder, and almond butter.
2. Blend on high until smooth and well combined.
3. If desired, add a few ice cubes and blend again until the shake reaches your desired consistency.
4. Pour into a glass and serve immediately.

Nutritional Information per serving:

Calories: 180 Protein: 20g Carbohydrates: 10g Fat: 8g Fiber: 4g

4. Strawberry Banana Oat Smoothie

Cook time: 5 minutes

Servings: 2

Ingredients:

- 1 cup unsweetened almond milk
- 1 cup frozen strawberries
- 1 small ripe banana
- 1/4 cup rolled oats
- 1 tablespoon honey or a natural sweetener (optional)

Instructions:

1. In a blender, combine the almond milk, frozen strawberries, ripe banana, rolled oats, and honey (if desired).
2. Blend on high until smooth and well combined.
3. Pour into glasses and serve immediately.

Nutritional Information per serving:

Calories: 120 Protein: 3g Carbohydrates: 25g Fat: 2g Fiber: 4g

CREATIVE EGG DISHES

5. Veggie Egg Muffins

Cook time: 25 minutes

Servings: 4

Ingredients:

- 6 large eggs
- 1/4 cup skim milk
- 1/2 cup diced bell peppers (any color)
- 1/2 cup diced zucchini
- 1/2 cup diced tomatoes
- 1/4 cup chopped spinach
- Salt and pepper to taste

Instructions:

1. Preheat the oven to 350°F (175°C) and lightly grease a muffin tin.
2. In a bowl, whisk together the eggs, skim milk, salt, and pepper.
3. Stir in the diced bell peppers, zucchini, tomatoes, and chopped spinach.
4. Pour the egg mixture into the prepared muffin tin, filling each cup about 3/4 full.
5. Bake for 20-25 minutes, or until the egg muffins are set and slightly golden on top.
6. Remove from the oven and let them cool for a few minutes before serving.

Nutritional Information per serving (2 egg muffins):

Calories: 150 Protein: 14g Carbohydrates: 5g Fat: 8g Fiber: 1g

6. Spinach and Mushroom Egg White Omelet

Cook time: 15 minutes

Servings: 1

Ingredients:

- 4 egg whites
- 1 cup fresh spinach
- 1/2 cup sliced mushrooms
- 1/4 cup diced onion
- 1 clove garlic, minced
- Salt and pepper to taste
- Cooking spray

Instructions:

1. Heat a non-stick skillet over medium heat and spray with cooking spray.
2. Add the diced onion and minced garlic to the skillet and sauté until fragrant.
3. Add the sliced mushrooms and sauté until they start to soften.
4. Add the fresh spinach to the skillet and cook until wilted.
5. In a bowl, whisk the egg whites with salt and pepper.
6. Pour the whisked egg whites into the skillet, covering the vegetables.
7. Cook for a few minutes until the edges of the omelet start to set.
8. Carefully fold the omelet in half and cook for another minute or two, until the eggs are fully cooked.
9. Slide the omelet onto a plate and serve.

Nutritional Information per serving:

Calories: 120 Protein: 20g Carbohydrates: 6g Fat: 0g Fiber: 2g

7. Avocado Egg Salad

Cook time: 10 minutes

Servings: 2

Ingredients:

- 4 hard-boiled eggs, peeled and chopped
- 1 ripe avocado, mashed
- 2 tablespoons Greek yogurt
- 1 tablespoon lemon juice
- 1/4 cup diced red onion
- 1/4 cup diced celery
- Salt and pepper to taste
- Whole grain bread or lettuce leaves for serving

Instructions:

1. In a bowl, combine the chopped hard-boiled eggs, mashed avocado, Greek yogurt, lemon juice, diced red onion, and diced celery.
2. Mix well until all the ingredients are evenly incorporated.
3. Season with salt and pepper to taste.
4. Serve the avocado egg salad on whole grain bread as a sandwich or wrapped in lettuce leaves as a low-carb option.

Nutritional Information per serving (without bread):

Calories: 180 Protein: 13g Carbohydrates: 8g Fat: 12g Fiber: 5g

8. Zucchini Egg Cups

Cook time: 25 minutes

Servings: 4

Ingredients:

- 2 medium zucchini, grated
- 4 large eggs
- 1/4 cup grated Parmesan cheese
- 2 tablespoons chopped fresh herbs (such as basil or parsley)
- Salt and pepper to taste

Instructions:

1. Preheat the oven to 375°F (190°C) and grease a muffin tin.
2. Place the grated zucchini in a clean kitchen towel and squeeze out the excess moisture.
3. In a bowl, combine the grated zucchini, eggs, Parmesan cheese, chopped fresh herbs, salt, and pepper.
4. Divide the mixture evenly among the cups of the greased muffin tin.
5. Bake for 20-25 minutes, or until the egg cups are set and slightly golden on top.
6. Remove from the oven and let them cool for a few minutes before serving.

Nutritional Information per serving (2 egg cups):

Calories: 100 Protein: 9g Carbohydrates: 4g Fat: 6g Fiber: 1g

HEALTHY CEREAL AND GRANOLA OPTIONS

9. Chia Seed Pudding with Fresh Berries

Preparation time: 5 minutes (+ 4 hours chilling time)

Servings: 2

Ingredients:

- 1/4 cup chia seeds
- 1 cup unsweetened almond milk
- 1 tablespoon honey or a natural sweetener
- 1/2 teaspoon vanilla extract
- Fresh berries (such as strawberries, blueberries, raspberries) for topping

Instructions:

1. In a bowl, combine the chia seeds, almond milk, honey, and vanilla extract. Stir well to evenly distribute the chia seeds.
2. Cover the bowl and refrigerate for at least 4 hours or overnight, allowing the chia seeds to absorb the liquid and create a pudding-like consistency.
3. Once the chia pudding has set, give it a good stir to break up any clumps.
4. Divide the pudding into serving bowls or jars and top with fresh berries.
5. Serve chilled.

Nutritional Information per serving:

Calories: 150 Protein: 5g Carbohydrates: 17g Fat: 7g Fiber: 10g

10. Yogurt Parfait with Homemade Granola

Preparation time: 5 minutes

Servings: 1

Ingredients:

- 1/2 cup Greek yogurt
- 1/4 cup homemade granola (see Recipe 1)
- 1/4 cup fresh mixed berries (such as strawberries, blueberries, raspberries)
- 1 tablespoon honey or a natural sweetener (optional)

Instructions:

1. In a glass or bowl, layer half of the Greek yogurt.
2. Sprinkle half of the homemade granola over the yogurt.
3. Add half of the fresh mixed berries on top.
4. Repeat the layers with the remaining yogurt, granola, and berries.
5. Drizzle with honey, if desired, for extra sweetness.
6. Serve immediately.

Nutritional Information per serving:

Calories: 180 Protein: 13g Carbohydrates: 23g Fat: 6g Fiber: 4g

11. Coconut Almond Granola Bars

Cook time: 20 minutes (+ chilling time)

Servings: 8

Ingredients:

- 1 1/2 cups old-fashioned rolled oats
- 1/2 cup unsweetened shredded coconut
- 1/4 cup chopped almonds
- 2 tablespoons almond butter
- 2 tablespoons honey or a natural sweetener
- 1 tablespoon coconut oil, melted
- 1/2 teaspoon vanilla extract
- Pinch of salt
- 1/4 cup mini dark chocolate chips (optional)

Instructions:

1. Preheat the oven to 350°F (175°C) and line a square baking pan with parchment paper.
2. In a large bowl, combine the rolled oats, shredded coconut, chopped almonds, almond butter, honey, melted coconut oil, vanilla extract, salt, and mini dark chocolate chips (if using). Mix well until all the ingredients are evenly combined.
3. Press the mixture firmly into the prepared baking pan, ensuring it is evenly spread and tightly packed.
4. Bake for 15-20 minutes, or until the edges are golden brown.
5. Remove from the oven and let it cool completely in the pan.
6. Once cooled, transfer the pan to the refrigerator and chill for at least 2 hours to allow the granola bars to firm up.
7. Cut into bars and serve.

Nutritional Information per serving (1 bar):

Calories: 160 Protein: 4g Carbohydrates: 18g Fat: 9g Fiber: 3g

12. Quinoa Breakfast Bowl

Cook time: 20 minutes

Servings: 2

Ingredients:

- 1/2 cup cooked quinoa
- 1 cup unsweetened almond milk
- 1 tablespoon honey or a natural sweetener
- 1/2 teaspoon vanilla extract
- 1/4 teaspoon ground cinnamon
- 1/4 cup sliced almonds
- 1/4 cup fresh mixed berries (such as strawberries, blueberries, raspberries)

Instructions:

1. In a small saucepan, combine the cooked quinoa, almond milk, honey, vanilla extract, and ground cinnamon.
2. Cook over medium heat, stirring occasionally, until the mixture comes to a gentle boil.
3. Reduce the heat to low and simmer for 10-15 minutes, or until the quinoa absorbs most of the liquid and reaches a creamy consistency.
4. Remove from heat and let it cool for a few minutes.
5. Divide the quinoa mixture into serving bowls and top with sliced almonds and fresh mixed berries.
6. Serve warm.

Nutritional Information per serving:

Calories: 180 Protein: 6g Carbohydrates: 25g Fat: 6g Fiber: 4g

CHAPTER 4

LUNCHTIME FAVORITES

SATISFYING SALADS AND DRESSINGS

13.Spinach and Strawberry Salad

Preparation time: 10 minutes

Servings: 2

Ingredients:

- 4 cups baby spinach leaves
- 1 cup sliced strawberries
- 1/4 cup crumbled goat cheese
- 2 tablespoons chopped walnuts
- 2 tablespoons balsamic vinegar
- 1 tablespoon extra virgin olive oil
- 1 teaspoon honey or a natural sweetener

Instructions:

1. In a large bowl, combine the baby spinach leaves, sliced strawberries, crumbled goat cheese, and chopped walnuts.
2. In a small bowl, whisk together the balsamic vinegar, olive oil, and honey until well combined.
3. Drizzle the dressing over the salad and toss to coat all the ingredients.
4. Serve immediately.

Nutritional Information per serving:

Calories: 180 Protein: 6g Carbohydrates: 10g Fat: 14g Fiber: 3g

14. Grilled Chicken Caesar Salad

Cook time: 20 minutes

Servings: 2

Ingredients:

- 2 boneless, skinless chicken breasts
- 4 cups romaine lettuce, chopped
- 1/4 cup grated Parmesan cheese
- Whole wheat croutons (optional)
- Caesar dressing (see Recipe 6)
- Salt and pepper to taste

Instructions:

1. Preheat the grill or stovetop grill pan over medium-high heat.
2. Season the chicken breasts with salt and pepper.
3. Grill the chicken for 6-8 minutes per side, or until cooked through and no longer pink in the center.
4. Remove the chicken from the grill and let it rest for a few minutes.
5. Slice the grilled chicken into thin strips.
6. In a large bowl, combine the chopped romaine lettuce, grated Parmesan cheese, and whole wheat croutons (if using).
7. Drizzle with Caesar dressing and toss to coat the salad evenly.
8. Divide the salad into serving plates and top with the sliced grilled chicken.
9. Serve immediately.

Nutritional Information per serving:

Calories: 220 Protein: 30g Carbohydrates: 8g Fat: 7g Fiber: 3g

15. Asian Quinoa Salad

Cook time: 15 minutes

Servings: 4

Ingredients:

- 1 cup cooked quinoa
- 1 cup shredded red cabbage
- 1/2 cup grated carrots
- 1/2 cup chopped cucumber
- 1/4 cup chopped green onions
- 1/4 cup chopped cilantro
- 2 tablespoons low-sodium soy sauce
- 1 tablespoon rice vinegar
- 1 tablespoon sesame oil
- 1 teaspoon honey or a natural sweetener
- Sesame seeds for garnish (optional)

Instructions:

1. In a large bowl, combine the cooked quinoa, shredded red cabbage, grated carrots, chopped cucumber, green onions, and cilantro.
2. In a separate small bowl, whisk together the soy sauce, rice vinegar, sesame oil, and honey until well combined.
3. Pour the dressing over the quinoa salad and toss to coat all the ingredients.
4. Sprinkle with sesame seeds for garnish, if desired.
5. Serve chilled or at room temperature.

Nutritional Information per serving:

Calories: 160 Protein: 5g Carbohydrates: 21gFat: 6g Fiber: 4g

16. Mediterranean Chickpea Salad

Preparation time: 10 minutes

Servings: 4

Ingredients:

- 2 cups canned chickpeas, drained and rinsed
- 1 cup diced cucumber
- 1 cup cherry tomatoes, halved
- 1/2 cup diced red onion
- 1/4 cup chopped Kalamata olives
- 1/4 cup crumbled feta cheese
- 2 tablespoons fresh lemon juice
- 2 tablespoons extra virgin olive oil
- 1 tablespoon chopped fresh parsley
- Salt and pepper to taste

Instructions:

1. In a large bowl, combine the chickpeas, diced cucumber, cherry tomatoes, diced red onion, Kalamata olives, and crumbled feta cheese.
2. In a small bowl, whisk together the fresh lemon juice, olive oil, chopped parsley, salt, and pepper.
3. Pour the dressing over the chickpea salad and toss to coat all the ingredients.
4. Adjust the seasoning if needed.
5. Serve chilled.

Nutritional Information per serving:

Calories: 220 Protein: 9g Carbohydrates: 26g Fat: 9g Fiber: 8g

17. Veggie Hummus Wrap

Preparation time: 10 minutes

Servings: 2

Ingredients:

- 2 whole wheat tortilla wraps
- 1/2 cup hummus
- 1/2 cup baby spinach leaves
- 1/2 cup sliced bell peppers
- 1/4 cup sliced cucumber
- 1/4 cup shredded carrots
- Salt and pepper to taste

Instructions:

1. Lay the whole wheat tortilla wraps flat on a clean surface.
2. Spread hummus evenly over each wrap.
3. Layer baby spinach leaves, sliced bell peppers, sliced cucumber, and shredded carrots on top of the hummus.
4. Season with salt and pepper.
5. Roll up the wraps tightly and cut them in half.
6. Serve immediately.

Nutritional Information per serving:

Calories: 200 Protein: 6g Carbohydrates: 28g Fat: 8g Fiber: 7g

18. Turkey and Avocado Sandwich

Preparation time: 10 minutes

Servings: 2

Ingredients:

- 4 slices whole wheat bread
- 4 ounces sliced turkey breast
- 1/2 avocado, sliced
- 1/4 cup baby spinach leaves
- 2 tablespoons Dijon mustard
- Salt and pepper to taste

Instructions:

1. Place the whole wheat bread slices on a clean surface.
2. Spread Dijon mustard evenly on two slices of bread.
3. Layer sliced turkey breast, avocado slices, and baby spinach leaves on top of the mustard.
4. Season with salt and pepper.
5. Top with the remaining bread slices.
6. Cut the sandwiches diagonally in half.
7. Serve immediately.

Nutritional Information per serving:

Calories: 230 Protein: 16g Carbohydrates: 24g Fat: 9g Fiber: 6g

19. Greek Chicken Wrap

Cook time: 15 minutes

Servings: 2

Ingredients:

- 2 whole wheat tortilla wraps
- 8 ounces cooked chicken breast, sliced
- 1/4 cup sliced cucumber
- 1/4 cup diced tomatoes
- 1/4 cup diced red onion
- 2 tablespoons crumbled feta cheese
- 2 tablespoons Greek yogurt
- 1 tablespoon fresh lemon juice
- 1/2 teaspoon dried oregano
- Salt and pepper to taste

Instructions:

1. In a small bowl, combine Greek yogurt, fresh lemon juice, dried oregano, salt, and pepper. Stir well to make the dressing.
2. Lay the whole wheat tortilla wraps flat on a clean surface.
3. Spread the Greek yogurt dressing evenly over each wrap.
4. Layer sliced chicken breast, sliced cucumber, diced tomatoes, diced red onion, and crumbled feta cheese on top of the dressing.
5. Roll up the wraps tightly and cut them in half.
6. Serve immediately.

Nutritional Information per serving:

Calories: 250 Protein: 28g Carbohydrates: 19g Fat: 7g Fiber: 4g

20. Caprese Sandwich

Preparation time: 10 minutes

Servings: 2

Ingredients:

- 4 slices whole wheat bread
- 4 slices fresh mozzarella cheese
- 1 cup sliced tomatoes
- 1/4 cup fresh basil leaves
- 1 tablespoon balsamic glaze
- Salt and pepper to taste

Instructions:

1. Place the whole wheat bread slices on a clean surface.
2. Layer fresh mozzarella cheese slices, sliced tomatoes, and fresh basil leaves on two slices of bread.
3. Season with salt and pepper.
4. Drizzle balsamic glaze over the filling.
5. Top with the remaining bread slices.
6. Cut the sandwiches diagonally in half.
7. Serve immediately.

Nutritional Information per serving:

Calories: 220 Protein: 15g Carbohydrates: 23g Fat: 8g Fiber: 4g

21. Vegetable Lentil Soup

Preparation time: 10 minutes

Cook time: 30 minutes

Servings: 4

Ingredients:

- 1 tablespoon olive oil
- 1 onion, chopped
- 2 carrots, diced
- 2 celery stalks, diced
- 2 cloves garlic, minced
- 1 cup dried lentils
- 4 cups vegetable broth
- 1 can (14 ounces) diced tomatoes
- 1 teaspoon ground cumin
- 1 teaspoon dried thyme
- Salt and pepper to taste

Instructions:

1. In a large pot, heat olive oil over medium heat.
2. Add onion, carrots, celery, and garlic. Sauté until the vegetables are tender.
3. Add dried lentils, vegetable broth, diced tomatoes, ground cumin, dried thyme, salt, and pepper to the pot. Bring the mixture to a boil, then reduce the heat to low.
4. Cover the pot and simmer for about 30 minutes, or until the lentils are cooked and tender.
5. Adjust the seasoning if needed. Serve hot.

Nutritional Information per serving:

Calories: 220 Protein: 14g Carbohydrates: 40g Fat: 2g Fiber: 15g

22. Chicken and Vegetable Stew

Preparation time: 15 minutes

Cook time: 40 minutes

Servings: 4

Ingredients:

- 1 tablespoon olive oil
- 1 onion, chopped
- 2 carrots, diced
- 2 celery stalks, diced
- 2 cloves garlic, minced
- 2 boneless, skinless chicken breasts, cut into bite-sized pieces
- 4 cups chicken broth
- 1 can (14 ounces) diced tomatoes
- 1 teaspoon dried thyme
- 1/2 teaspoon paprika
- Salt and pepper to taste

Instructions:

1. In a large pot, heat olive oil over medium heat.
2. Add onion, carrots, celery, and garlic. Sauté until the vegetables are tender.
3. Add chicken pieces to the pot and cook until they are no longer pink.
4. Pour in chicken broth, diced tomatoes, dried thyme, paprika, salt, and pepper.
5. Bring the mixture to a boil, then reduce the heat to low.
6. Cover the pot and simmer for about 40 minutes, or until the chicken is cooked through and the flavors have melded together.
7. Adjust the seasoning if needed. Serve hot.

Nutritional Information per serving:

Calories: 250 Protein: 24g Carbohydrates: 20g Fat: 6g Fiber: 4g

23. Butternut Squash Soup

Preparation time: 15 minutes

Cook time: 40 minutes

Servings: 4

Ingredients:

- 1 butternut squash, peeled, seeded, and cubed
- 1 onion, chopped
- 2 carrots, diced
- 2 cloves garlic, minced
- 4 cups vegetable broth
- 1/2 teaspoon ground cinnamon
- 1/4 teaspoon ground nutmeg
- Salt and pepper to taste

Instructions:

1. In a large pot, combine butternut squash, onion, carrots, garlic, and vegetable broth.
2. Bring the mixture to a boil, then reduce the heat to low.
3. Cover the pot and simmer for about 40 minutes, or until the butternut squash is tender.
4. Use an immersion blender or a regular blender to puree the soup until smooth.
5. Stir in ground cinnamon, ground nutmeg, salt, and pepper.
6. Adjust the seasoning if needed.
7. Serve hot.

Nutritional Information per serving:

Calories: 180 Protein: 3g Carbohydrates: 42g Fat: 1g Fiber: 7g

24. Minestrone Soup

Preparation time: 15 minutes

Cook time: 40 minutes

Servings: 4

Ingredients:

- 1 tablespoon olive oil
- 1 onion, chopped
- 2 carrots, diced
- 2 celery stalks, diced
- 2 cloves garlic, minced
- 4 cups vegetable broth
- 1 can (14 ounces) diced tomatoes
- 1 can (15 ounces) kidney beans, drained and rinsed
- 1/2 cup small pasta (such as elbow or ditalini)
- 1 teaspoon dried basil
- 1 teaspoon dried oregano
- Salt and pepper to taste

Instructions:

1. In a large pot, heat olive oil over medium heat.
2. Add onion, carrots, celery, and garlic. Sauté until the vegetables are tender.
3. Add vegetable broth, diced tomatoes, kidney beans, small pasta, dried basil, dried oregano, salt, and pepper to the pot. Bring the mixture to a boil, then reduce the heat to low.
4. Cover the pot and simmer for about 40 minutes, or until the pasta is cooked al dente and the flavors have melded together.
5. Adjust the seasoning if needed. Serve hot.

Nutritional Information per serving:

Calories: 220 Protein: 10g Carbohydrates: 42g Fat: 2g Fiber: 10g

CHAPTER 5

DINNER DELICACIES

FLAVORFUL AND LEAN PROTEIN OPTIONS

25. Baked Salmon with Lemon Dill Sauce

Preparation time: 10 minutes

Cook time: 15 minutes

Servings: 4

Ingredients:

- 4 salmon fillets
- 2 tablespoons lemon juice
- 1 tablespoon olive oil
- 2 cloves garlic, minced
- 1 tablespoon chopped fresh dill
- Salt and pepper to taste

Instructions:

1. Preheat the oven to 400°F (200°C).
2. In a small bowl, whisk together lemon juice, olive oil, minced garlic, chopped fresh dill, salt, and pepper. Place salmon fillets on a baking sheet lined with parchment paper.
3. Pour the lemon dill sauce over the salmon, making sure it is evenly coated.
4. Bake the salmon for about 15 minutes, or until it is cooked through and flakes easily with a fork.
5. Remove the salmon from the oven and let it rest for a few minutes before serving. Serve hot.

Nutritional Information per serving:

Calories: 250 Protein: 28g Carbohydrates: 1g Fat: 15g Fiber: 0g

26. Grilled Lemon Herb Chicken

Preparation time: 10 minutes

Cook time: 20 minutes

Servings: 4

Ingredients:

- 4 boneless, skinless chicken breasts
- 2 tablespoons lemon juice
- 1 tablespoon olive oil
- 2 cloves garlic, minced
- 1 teaspoon dried thyme
- 1 teaspoon dried rosemary
- Salt and pepper to taste

Instructions:

1. In a small bowl, whisk together lemon juice, olive oil, minced garlic, dried thyme, dried rosemary, salt, and pepper.
2. Place chicken breasts in a shallow dish and pour the marinade over them. Make sure the chicken is evenly coated. Let it marinate for 15 minutes.
3. Preheat the grill to medium-high heat.
4. Grill the chicken for about 10 minutes on each side, or until the internal temperature reaches 165°F (74°C).
5. Remove the chicken from the grill and let it rest for a few minutes before serving.
6. Serve hot.

Nutritional Information per serving:

Calories: 180 Protein: 30g Carbohydrates: 1g Fat: 6g Fiber: 0g

27. Grilled Balsamic Glazed Pork Tenderloin

Preparation time: 10 minutes

Cook time: 25 minutes

Servings: 4

Ingredients:

- 1 pound pork tenderloin
- 2 tablespoons balsamic vinegar
- 1 tablespoon olive oil
- 1 tablespoon Dijon mustard
- 1 clove garlic, minced
- 1 teaspoon dried thyme
- Salt and pepper to taste

Instructions:

1. Preheat the grill to medium-high heat.
2. In a small bowl, whisk together balsamic vinegar, olive oil, Dijon mustard, minced garlic, dried thyme, salt, and pepper.
3. Place the pork tenderloin on the grill and brush the balsamic glaze over it.
4. Grill the pork for about 20-25 minutes, turning occasionally and brushing with the glaze, until the internal temperature reaches 145°F (63°C).
5. Remove the pork from the grill and let it rest for a few minutes before slicing.
6. Serve hot.

Nutritional Information per serving:

Calories: 200 Protein: 28g Carbohydrates: 2g Fat: 8g Fiber: 0g

28. Teriyaki Turkey Meatballs

Preparation time: 15 minutes

Cook time: 25 minutes

Servings: 4

Ingredients:

- 1 pound lean ground turkey
- 1/4 cup whole wheat breadcrumbs
- 2 tablespoons low-sodium soy sauce
- 1 tablespoon honey
- 1 clove garlic, minced
- 1 teaspoon grated fresh ginger
- 1 green onion, thinly sliced
- Sesame seeds for garnish (optional)

Instructions:

1. Preheat the oven to 375°F (190°C).
2. In a large bowl, combine ground turkey, whole wheat breadcrumbs, low-sodium soy sauce, honey, minced garlic, grated ginger, and sliced green onion. Mix well to combine.
3. Shape the mixture into meatballs, approximately 1 inch in diameter.
4. Place the meatballs on a baking sheet lined with parchment paper.
5. Bake the meatballs for about 20-25 minutes, or until they are cooked through and browned.
6. Remove the meatballs from the oven and let them cool slightly.
7. Sprinkle sesame seeds on top for garnish, if desired.
8. Serve hot.

Nutritional Information per serving:

Calories: 170 Protein: 20g Carbohydrates: 6g Fat: 7g Fiber: 1g

29. Lemon Garlic Shrimp Stir-Fry

Preparation time: 10 minutes

Cook time: 10 minutes

Servings: 4

Ingredients:

- 1 pound shrimp, peeled and deveined
- 2 tablespoons lemon juice
- 2 cloves garlic, minced
- 1 tablespoon low-sodium soy sauce
- 1 tablespoon olive oil
- 1 teaspoon cornstarch
- 1/2 teaspoon red pepper flakes (optional)
- Salt and pepper to taste
- Sliced green onions for garnish

Instructions:

1. In a small bowl, whisk together lemon juice, minced garlic, low-sodium soy sauce, olive oil, cornstarch, red pepper flakes (if using), salt, and pepper.
2. Heat a large skillet or wok over medium-high heat.
3. Add the shrimp to the skillet and pour the lemon garlic sauce over them.
4. Stir-fry the shrimp for about 5-6 minutes, or until they are cooked through and pink.
5. Remove the skillet from the heat.
6. Garnish with sliced green onions.
7. Serve hot.

Nutritional Information per serving:

Calories: 160 Protein: 24g Carbohydrates: 3g Fat: 6g Fiber: 0g

30. Baked Cod with Herbed Yogurt Sauce

Preparation time: 10 minutes

Cook time: 20 minutes

Servings: 4

Ingredients:

- 4 cod fillets
- 1/2 cup plain Greek yogurt
- 1 tablespoon chopped fresh dill
- 1 tablespoon chopped fresh parsley
- 1 tablespoon lemon juice
- 1 clove garlic, minced
- Salt and pepper to taste

Instructions:

1. Preheat the oven to 400°F (200°C).
2. In a small bowl, combine plain Greek yogurt, chopped fresh dill, chopped fresh parsley, lemon juice, minced garlic, salt, and pepper. Mix well to make the herbed yogurt sauce.
3. Place cod fillets on a baking sheet lined with parchment paper.
4. Spread the herbed yogurt sauce evenly over the top of each cod fillet.
5. Bake the cod for about 15-20 minutes, or until it is cooked through and flakes easily with a fork.
6. Remove the cod from the oven and let it rest for a few minutes before serving.
7. Serve hot.

Nutritional Information per serving:

Calories: 150 Protein: 25g Carbohydrates: 3g Fat: 3g Fiber: 0g

COLORFUL VEGGIE CREATIONS

31. Zucchini Noodles with Tomato Basil Sauce

Preparation time: 15 minutes

Cook time: 15 minutes

Servings: 4

Ingredients:

- 4 medium zucchini
- 2 cups cherry tomatoes, halved
- 2 cloves garlic, minced
- 2 tablespoons olive oil
- 1/4 cup chopped fresh basil
- 1/4 teaspoon red pepper flakes (optional)
- Salt and pepper to taste
- Grated Parmesan cheese for garnish (optional)

Instructions:

1. Spiralize the zucchini into noodles using a spiralizer or julienne peeler.
2. Heat olive oil in a large skillet over medium heat.
3. Add minced garlic and red pepper flakes (if using) to the skillet. Sauté for about 1 minute until fragrant.
4. Add cherry tomatoes to the skillet and cook for about 5 minutes until they start to soften.
5. Add zucchini noodles to the skillet and toss to coat them with the tomato mixture.
6. Cook for about 3-4 minutes, or until the zucchini noodles are tender but still crisp.
7. Stir in chopped fresh basil and season with salt and pepper.
8. Remove from heat and garnish with grated Parmesan cheese if desired.
9. Serve hot.

Nutritional Information per serving:

Calories: 80 Protein: 3g Carbohydrates: 8g Fat: 5g Fiber: 3g

32. Rainbow Veggie Stir-Fry

Preparation time: 10 minutes

Cook time: 15 minutes

Servings: 4

Ingredients:

- 1 red bell pepper, sliced
- 1 yellow bell pepper, sliced
- 1 green bell pepper, sliced
- 1 small zucchini, sliced
- 1 small yellow squash, sliced
- 1 cup broccoli florets
- 1 cup snap peas
- 2 cloves garlic, minced
- 2 tablespoons low-sodium soy sauce
- 1 tablespoon sesame oil
- 1 teaspoon grated fresh ginger
- Salt and pepper to taste

Instructions:

1. Heat sesame oil in a large skillet or wok over medium-high heat.
2. Add minced garlic and grated ginger to the skillet. Sauté for about 1 minute until fragrant.
3. Add bell peppers, zucchini, yellow squash, broccoli, and snap peas to the skillet. Stir-fry for about 5-7 minutes, or until the vegetables are crisp-tender.
4. Stir in low-sodium soy sauce and season with salt and pepper.
5. Cook for another 2-3 minutes, stirring occasionally.
6. Remove from heat and serve hot.

Nutritional Information per serving:

Calories: 100 Protein: 4g Carbohydrates: 12g Fat: 4g Fiber: 4g

33. Stuffed Bell Peppers

Preparation time: 20 minutes

Cook time: 25 minutes

Servings: 4

Ingredients:

- 4 bell peppers (any color), tops removed and seeded
- 1 cup cooked quinoa
- 1 cup black beans, drained and rinsed
- 1 cup corn kernels
- 1/2 cup diced tomatoes
- 1/2 cup diced red onion
- 1/4 cup chopped fresh cilantro
- 1 tablespoon olive oil
- 1 tablespoon lime juice
- 1 teaspoon ground cumin
- 1/2 teaspoon chili powder
- Salt and pepper to taste

Instructions:

1. Preheat the oven to 375°F (190°C).
2. In a large bowl, combine cooked quinoa, black beans, corn kernels, diced tomatoes, diced red onion, chopped fresh cilantro, olive oil, lime juice, ground cumin, chili powder, salt, and pepper. Mix well to combine.
3. Stuff each bell pepper with the quinoa mixture. Place the stuffed bell peppers in a baking dish.
4. Bake for about 25 minutes, or until the bell peppers are tender and the filling is heated through.
5. Remove from the oven and let them cool slightly before serving. Serve hot.

Nutritional Information per serving:

Calories: 180 Protein: 8g Carbohydrates: 30g Fat: 4g Fiber: 8g

34. Sweet Potato and Black Bean Tacos

Preparation time: 10 minutes

Cook time: 30 minutes

Servings: 4

Ingredients:

- 2 medium sweet potatoes, peeled and cubed
- 1 can black beans, drained and rinsed
- 1 red onion, sliced
- 1 red bell pepper, sliced
- 2 cloves garlic, minced
- 2 tablespoons olive oil
- 1 teaspoon ground cumin
- 1 teaspoon chili powder
- Corn tortillas
- Fresh cilantro for garnish

Instructions:

1. Preheat the oven to 400°F (200°C).
2. In a large bowl, toss sweet potato cubes with olive oil, ground cumin, chili powder, salt, and pepper.
3. Spread the seasoned sweet potatoes on a baking sheet and roast for about 25-30 minutes, or until they are tender and slightly caramelized. In a separate skillet, heat olive oil over medium heat.
4. Add sliced red onion, red bell pepper, and minced garlic to the skillet. Sauté for about 5-7 minutes, or until the vegetables are softened. Add black beans to the skillet and cook for another 2-3 minutes to heat through. Warm corn tortillas on a separate skillet or in the oven.
5. Assemble the tacos by filling each tortilla with roasted sweet potatoes, black bean mixture, and garnish with fresh cilantro. Serve

Nutritional Information per serving:

Calories: 220 Protein: 6g Carbohydrates: 40g Fat: 5g Fiber: 8g

35. Quinoa Stuffed Bell Peppers

Preparation time: 15 minutes

Cook time: 30 minutes

Servings: 4

Ingredients:

- 4 bell peppers (any color), tops removed and seeded
- 1 cup cooked quinoa
- 1 cup black beans, drained and rinsed
- 1 cup corn kernels
- 1/2 cup diced tomatoes
- 1/4 cup chopped fresh cilantro
- 1 tablespoon olive oil
- 1 tablespoon lime juice
- 1 teaspoon ground cumin
- 1/2 teaspoon chili powder
- Salt and pepper to taste

Instructions:

1. Preheat the oven to 375°F (190°C).
2. In a large bowl, combine cooked quinoa, black beans, corn kernels, diced tomatoes, chopped fresh cilantro, olive oil, lime juice, ground cumin, chili powder, salt, and pepper. Mix well to combine. Stuff each bell pepper with the quinoa mixture. Place the stuffed bell peppers in a baking dish.
3. Bake for about 25-30 minutes, or until the bell peppers are tender and the filling is heated through.
4. Remove from the oven and let them cool slightly before serving.

Nutritional Information per serving:

Calories: 200 Protein: 9g Carbohydrates: 38g Fat: 3g Fiber: 9g

36. Brown Rice and Vegetable Stir-Fry

Preparation time: 10 minutes

Cook time: 20 minutes

Servings: 4

Ingredients:

- 2 cups cooked brown rice
- 1 cup broccoli florets
- 1 cup snap peas
- 1 carrot, thinly sliced
- 1 red bell pepper, sliced
- 1 small onion, sliced
- 2 cloves garlic, minced
- 2 tablespoons low-sodium soy sauce
- 1 tablespoon sesame oil
- 1 tablespoon rice vinegar
- 1 teaspoon grated fresh ginger
- Salt and pepper to taste

Instructions:

1. Heat sesame oil in a large skillet or wok over medium-high heat.
2. Add minced garlic and grated ginger to the skillet. Sauté for about 1 minute until fragrant.
3. Add broccoli florets, snap peas, carrot slices, red bell pepper slices, and onion slices to the skillet. Stir-fry for about 5-7 minutes, or until the vegetables are crisp-tender.
4. In a small bowl, whisk together low-sodium soy sauce, rice vinegar, salt, and pepper.
5. Add cooked brown rice and the sauce mixture to the skillet. Stir well to combine and heat through.
6. Remove from heat and serve hot.

Nutritional Information per serving:

Calories: 230 Protein: 5g Carbohydrates: 40g Fat: 6g Fiber: 5g

37. Quinoa and Vegetable Stir-Fry

Preparation time: 10 minutes

Cook time: 20 minutes

Servings: 4

Ingredients:

- 1 cup cooked quinoa
- 1 cup broccoli florets
- 1 cup snap peas
- 1 carrot, thinly sliced
- 1 red bell pepper, sliced
- 1 small onion, sliced
- 2 cloves garlic, minced
- 2 tablespoons low-sodium soy sauce
- 1 tablespoon sesame oil
- 1 tablespoon rice vinegar
- 1 teaspoon grated fresh ginger
- Salt and pepper to taste

Instructions:

1. Heat sesame oil in a large skillet or wok over medium-high heat.
2. Add minced garlic and grated ginger to the skillet. Sauté for about 1 minute until fragrant.
3. Add broccoli florets, snap peas, carrot slices, red bell pepper slices, and onion slices to the skillet. Stir-fry for about 5-7 minutes, or until the vegetables are crisp-tender.
4. In a small bowl, whisk together low-sodium soy sauce, rice vinegar, salt, and pepper.
5. Add cooked quinoa and the sauce mixture to the skillet. Stir well to combine and heat through.
6. Remove from heat and serve hot.

Nutritional Information per serving:

Calories: 220 Protein: 7g Carbohydrates: 37g Fat: 6g Fiber: 6g

38. Whole Wheat Pasta with Roasted Vegetables

Preparation time: 10 minutes

Cook time: 30 minutes

Servings: 4

Ingredients:

- 8 ounces whole wheat pasta
- 1 small eggplant, diced
- 1 zucchini, diced
- 1 red bell pepper, sliced
- 1 small onion, sliced
- 2 cloves garlic, minced
- 2 tablespoons olive oil
- 1 teaspoon dried basil
- 1 teaspoon dried oregano
- Salt and pepper to taste
- Grated Parmesan cheese for garnish

Instructions:

1. Preheat the oven to 400°F (200°C).
2. In a large baking dish, toss together diced eggplant, diced zucchini, sliced red bell pepper, sliced onion, minced garlic, olive oil, dried basil, dried oregano, salt, and pepper.
3. Roast the vegetables in the preheated oven for about 25-30 minutes, or until they are tender and lightly browned. Meanwhile, cook the whole wheat pasta according to package instructions until al dente.
4. Drain the cooked pasta and transfer it to a serving dish.
5. Add the roasted vegetables to the pasta and toss gently to combine. Adjust seasoning if needed.
6. Serve the whole wheat pasta with roasted vegetables garnished with grated Parmesan cheese.

Nutritional Information per serving:

Calories: 280 Protein: 9g Carbohydrates: 48g Fat: 8g Fiber: 9g

CHAPTER 6

SNACKS AND TREATS

GUILT-FREE SNACK IDEAS

39. Baked Sweet Potato Chips

Cook time: 25 minutes

Servings: 2

Ingredients:

- 1 large sweet potato
- 1 tablespoon olive oil
- Salt and pepper to taste

Instructions:

1. Preheat the oven to 375°F (190°C) and line a baking sheet with parchment paper.
2. Slice the sweet potato into thin, even rounds.
3. In a bowl, toss the sweet potato slices with olive oil, salt, and pepper until coated evenly.
4. Arrange the slices in a single layer on the prepared baking sheet.
5. Bake for about 20-25 minutes, flipping halfway through, until the chips are crispy and golden.
6. Remove from the oven and let them cool before serving.

Nutritional Information per serving:

Calories: 100 Protein: 2g Carbohydrates: 18g Fat: 3g Fiber: 3g

40. Greek Yogurt and Berry Parfait

Preparation time: 5 minutes

Servings: 1

Ingredients:

- 1/2 cup non-fat Greek yogurt
- 1/4 cup mixed berries (strawberries, blueberries, raspberries)
- 1 tablespoon honey or stevia (optional)
- 1 tablespoon chopped nuts (e.g., almonds, walnuts)

Instructions:

1. In a glass or bowl, layer half of the Greek yogurt.
2. Top with half of the mixed berries.
3. Repeat the layers with the remaining yogurt and berries.
4. Drizzle with honey or sprinkle with stevia if desired.
5. Garnish with chopped nuts.
6. Enjoy immediately.

Nutritional Information per serving:

Calories: 150 Protein: 15g Carbohydrates: 20g Fat: 2g Fiber: 3g

41. Cucumber and Hummus Bites

Preparation time: 10 minutes

Servings: 2

Ingredients:

- 1 large cucumber
- 4 tablespoons hummus (flavor of your choice)
- Fresh dill or parsley for garnish

Instructions:

1. Slice the cucumber into thick rounds.
2. Using a spoon or knife, create a small indentation in the center of each cucumber round.
3. Fill each indentation with a teaspoon of hummus.
4. Garnish with fresh dill or parsley.
5. Serve as a refreshing snack.

Nutritional Information per serving:

Calories: 60 Protein: 2g Carbohydrates: 8g Fat: 3g Fiber: 2g

42. Veggie Sticks with Yogurt Dip

Preparation time: 10 minutes

Servings: 2

Ingredients:

- 2 medium carrots, cut into sticks
- 2 medium celery stalks, cut into sticks
- 1/2 cup non-fat Greek yogurt
- 1 tablespoon lemon juice
- 1/2 teaspoon dried dill
- Salt and pepper to taste

Instructions:

1. In a small bowl, combine Greek yogurt, lemon juice, dried dill, salt, and pepper. Mix well to make the dip.
2. Serve the carrot and celery sticks alongside the yogurt dip.

Nutritional Information per serving:

Calories: 50 Protein: 4g Carbohydrates: 8g Fat: 0g Fiber: 2g

43. Rice Cake with Avocado and Sliced Tomato

Preparation time: 5 minutes

Servings: 1

Ingredients:

- 1 rice cake
- 1/4 avocado, mashed
- 2-3 slices of tomato
- Salt and pepper to taste
- Fresh basil or cilantro for garnish

Instructions:

1. Spread the mashed avocado evenly on the rice cake.
2. Top with sliced tomato.
3. Season with salt and pepper.
4. Garnish with fresh basil or cilantro.
5. Enjoy as a light and satisfying snack.

Nutritional Information per serving:

Calories: 80 Protein: 2g Carbohydrates: 12g Fat: 4gFiber: 2g

44. Baked Zucchini Fries

Cook time: 25 minutes

Servings: 2

Ingredients:

- 2 medium zucchini, cut into sticks
- 1/4 cup whole wheat breadcrumbs
- 1/4 cup grated Parmesan cheese
- 1/2 teaspoon garlic powder
- 1/2 teaspoon dried oregano
- Salt and pepper to taste
- 1 large egg, beaten

Instructions:

1. Preheat the oven to 425°F (220°C) and line a baking sheet with parchment paper.
2. In a shallow bowl, combine breadcrumbs, grated Parmesan cheese, garlic powder, dried oregano, salt, and pepper.
3. Dip each zucchini stick into the beaten egg, then roll it in the breadcrumb mixture, pressing gently to adhere.
4. Place the coated zucchini sticks on the prepared baking sheet.
5. Bake for about 20-25 minutes, flipping halfway through, until the fries are golden and crispy.
6. Remove from the oven and let them cool slightly before serving.

Nutritional Information per serving:

Calories: 100 Protein: 7g Carbohydrates: 10g Fat: 4g Fiber: 3g

SWEET AND SAVORY TREATS

45. Baked Apple Chips

Cook time: 2 hours

Servings: 2

Ingredients:

- 2 apples (any variety)
- Cinnamon (optional)

Instructions:

1. Preheat the oven to 200°F (95°C) and line a baking sheet with parchment paper.
2. Wash and thinly slice the apples using a mandolin or a sharp knife.
3. Arrange the apple slices in a single layer on the prepared baking sheet.
4. Sprinkle with cinnamon if desired.
5. Bake for about 2 hours, or until the apple slices are crispy.
6. Allow them to cool completely before serving.

Nutritional Information per serving:

Calories: 50 Protein: 0g Carbohydrates: 14g Fat: 0g Fiber: 3g

46. Mini Caprese Skewers

Preparation time: 10 minutes

Servings: 2

Ingredients:

- 8 cherry tomatoes
- 8 mini mozzarella balls
- Fresh basil leaves
- Balsamic glaze (optional)
- Salt and pepper to taste

Instructions:

1. Skewer a cherry tomato, a mini mozzarella ball, and a fresh basil leaf onto toothpicks or skewers.
2. Repeat with the remaining ingredients.
3. Arrange the skewers on a serving plate.
4. Drizzle with balsamic glaze if desired.
5. Season with salt and pepper.
6. Serve as a delightful and satisfying snack.

Nutritional Information per serving:

Calories: 70 Protein: 4g Carbohydrates: 3g Fat: 5g Fiber: 1g

47. Chocolate Dipped Strawberries

Preparation time: 10 minutes

Chilling time: 30 minutes

Servings: 2

Ingredients:

- 10 strawberries
- 1 ounce dark chocolate (70% cocoa or higher)

Instructions:

1. Wash and pat dry the strawberries, leaving the stems intact.
2. In a microwave-safe bowl, melt the dark chocolate in short intervals, stirring in between until smooth.
3. Dip each strawberry into the melted chocolate, allowing any excess chocolate to drip off.
4. Place the chocolate-dipped strawberries on a parchment-lined tray.
5. Chill in the refrigerator for about 30 minutes, or until the chocolate is set.
6. Serve and enjoy as a guilt-free sweet treat.

Nutritional Information per serving:

Calories: 80 Protein: 2g Carbohydrates: 12g Fat: 4g Fiber: 3g

48. Baked Spiced Chickpeas

Cook time: 30 minutes

Servings: 2

Ingredients:

- 1 can (15 ounces) chickpeas, drained and rinsed
- 1 tablespoon olive oil
- 1/2 teaspoon paprika
- 1/2 teaspoon cumin
- 1/4 teaspoon garlic powder
- Salt and pepper to taste

Instructions:

1. Preheat the oven to 400°F (200°C) and line a baking sheet with parchment paper.
2. In a bowl, combine chickpeas, olive oil, paprika, cumin, garlic powder, salt, and pepper. Toss until the chickpeas are well coated.
3. Spread the chickpeas in a single layer on the prepared baking sheet.
4. Bake for about 25-30 minutes, or until the chickpeas are crispy and golden.
5. Remove from the oven and let them cool before serving.

Nutritional Information per serving:

Calories: 120 Protein: 5g Carbohydrates: 16g Fat: 4g Fiber: 4g

49. Cucumber Sushi Rolls

Preparation time: 15 minutes

Servings: 2

Ingredients:

- 2 large cucumbers
- 1 small carrot, julienned
- 1/2 avocado, sliced
- 1/4 cup cooked quinoa
- 2 tablespoons low-sodium soy sauce
- 1 tablespoon rice vinegar
- 1 teaspoon sesame seeds

Instructions:

1. Slice the cucumbers lengthwise into thin strips using a mandoline or a vegetable peeler.
2. Lay a cucumber strip flat and place a few julienned carrots, avocado slices, and a small amount of cooked quinoa on one end.
3. Roll the cucumber strip tightly, enclosing the filling, and secure with a toothpick if needed.
4. Repeat with the remaining cucumber strips and filling ingredients.
5. In a small bowl, mix the low-sodium soy sauce and rice vinegar to make a dipping sauce.
6. Sprinkle the sushi rolls with sesame seeds and serve with the dipping sauce.

Nutritional Information per serving:

Calories: 80 Protein: 3g Carbohydrates: 12g Fat: 3g Fiber: 4g

50. Baked Buffalo Cauliflower Bites

Cook time: 30 minutes

Servings: 2

Ingredients:

- 1 small head of cauliflower, cut into florets
- 1/4 cup whole wheat flour
- 1/4 cup unsweetened almond milk
- 1/4 cup buffalo sauce
- 1 tablespoon melted coconut oil
- 1/2 teaspoon garlic powder
- Salt and pepper to taste

Instructions:

1. Preheat the oven to 425°F (220°C) and line a baking sheet with parchment paper.
2. In a bowl, whisk together the whole wheat flour, almond milk, buffalo sauce, melted coconut oil, garlic powder, salt, and pepper until well combined.
3. Dip each cauliflower floret into the buffalo mixture, making sure it is coated evenly, and place it on the prepared baking sheet.
4. Bake for about 25-30 minutes, or until the cauliflower is tender and the coating is crispy.
5. Allow them to cool slightly before serving.

Nutritional Information per serving:

Calories: 90 Protein: 3g Carbohydrates: 12g Fat: 4g Fiber: 3g

CHAPTER 7

FREQUENTLY ASKED QUESTIONS

CAN I BUILD MUSCLE ON A CALORIE DEFICIT?

Answer: While it's challenging to build significant muscle mass in a calorie deficit, it is possible to maintain and even build some muscle with the right approach. Adequate protein intake, resistance training, and strategic meal timing can help preserve muscle while in a calorie deficit.

HOW LONG SHOULD I STAY IN A CALORIE DEFICIT?

Answer: The duration of a calorie deficit depends on your individual goals, current weight, and overall health. It's generally recommended to aim for a gradual and sustainable weight loss of 1-2 pounds per week. Consulting with a healthcare professional or registered dietitian can help determine the appropriate duration for your specific needs.

IS CALORIE COUNTING NECESSARY?

Answer: While calorie counting can be a helpful tool for managing your calorie intake, it is not essential for everyone. Some individuals may prefer intuitive eating or following portion control guidelines. However, if you find it challenging to gauge portion sizes or control your calorie intake, counting calories can provide valuable information and help you stay within your calorie deficit goals.

HOW CAN I MANAGE HUNGER WHILE IN A CALORIE DEFICIT?

Answer: Managing hunger while in a calorie deficit can be a common challenge. To combat hunger, focus on consuming high-fiber foods, lean proteins, and healthy fats that provide satiety. Drinking plenty of water, eating balanced meals, and including filling foods like fruits, vegetables, and whole grains can help you feel fuller for longer.

IS IT SAFE TO STAY IN A CALORIE DEFICIT FOR AN EXTENDED PERIOD?

Answer: While short-term calorie deficits are generally safe and effective for weight loss, prolonged or extreme calorie deficits can have negative health consequences. It is important to prioritize your overall well-being and ensure you are meeting your nutritional needs. If you plan to stay in a calorie deficit for an extended period, it is advisable to consult with a healthcare professional or registered dietitian to ensure you are maintaining a balanced and sustainable approach.

HOW CAN I OVERCOME PLATEAUS IN A CALORIE DEFICIT?

Answer: Plateaus can occur during a calorie deficit when weight loss stalls. To overcome plateaus, consider adjusting your calorie intake or increasing physical activity. Incorporating resistance training can help build muscle and boost your metabolism. Additionally, be patient and stay consistent, as weight loss progress may vary and plateaus are a normal part of the process.

2 WEEK MEAL PLAN

WEEK 1

DAY	BREAKFAST	LUNCH	DINNER	SNACK
Day 1	Scrambled Eggs with Veggies	Chicken and Quinoa Salad	Baked Salmon with Asparagus	Greek Yogurt with Berries
Day 2	Oatmeal with Banana	Turkey Wrap	Grilled Chicken with Broccoli	Carrot Sticks with Hummus
Day 3	Green Smoothie	Veggie Stir-Fry with Tofu	Shrimp and Quinoa Stir-Fry	Almonds
Day 4	Greek Yogurt with Granola	Lentil Soup	Baked Cod with Roasted Vegetables	Apple Slices with Peanut Butter
Day 5	Protein Pancakes	Grilled Chicken Salad	Beef and Vegetable Stir-Fry	Cottage Cheese with Pineapple
Day 6	Avocado Toast	Quinoa and Chickpea Salad	Turkey Meatballs with Zucchini Noodles	Cucumber Slices with Guacamole
Day 7	Fruit Salad	Spinach and Feta Stuffed Chicken Breast	Grilled Steak with Steamed Vegetables	Mixed Berries

WEEK 2

DAY	BREAKFAST	LUNCH	DINNER	SNACK
Day 8	Scrambled Eggs with Spinach	Quinoa Salad	Baked Salmon with Green Beans	Greek Yogurt with Berries
Day 9	Berry Smoothie	Turkey Wrap	Grilled Chicken with Roasted Sweet Potatoes	Carrot Sticks with Hummus
Day 10	Overnight Chia Pudding	Veggie Stir-Fry with Chicken	Shrimp and Quinoa Salad	Almonds
Day 11	Whole Wheat Toast with Avocado	Lentil Soup	Baked Cod with Quinoa	Apple Slices with Peanut Butter
Day 12	Vegetable Omelet	Chicken Caesar Salad	Beef Stir-Fry with Brown Rice	Cottage Cheese with Pineapple
Day 13	Banana Pancakes	Quinoa and Black Bean Salad	Turkey and Vegetable Skewers	Cucumber Slices with Guacamole
Day 14	Yogurt Parfait	Spinach Salad	Grilled Tofu with Stir-Fried Veggies	Mixed Berries

CONCLUSION

Congratulations on reaching the end of this culinary journey! As we close the chapter on the Calorie Deficit Cookbook, I want to take a moment to reflect on the incredible strides you have made towards a healthier, more fulfilling lifestyle. You have shown dedication, courage, and a relentless commitment to your well-being, and I couldn't be prouder of you.

Throughout these pages, we have explored the transformative power of calorie deficit cooking and the boundless possibilities it offers. Together, we have discovered that healthy eating doesn't mean sacrificing flavor or satisfaction. It is about finding the delicate balance between nourishing our bodies and indulging our taste buds.

As you embraced the vibrant breakfast smoothies, savory wraps and sandwiches, nutritious soups and stews, and the myriad of other delectable recipes, you embarked on a culinary adventure that defied the limitations often associated with weight loss. You have come to realize that healthy eating is not a restrictive sentence but a gateway to a world of flavor, creativity, and personal empowerment.

But this is not where your journey ends; rather, it is just the beginning. The Calorie Deficit Cookbook has provided you with a solid foundation, equipping you with the knowledge, tools, and recipes to continue crafting your own path to wellness. The recipes within these pages have nurtured your body, nourished your soul, and fostered a newfound appreciation for the art of cooking and eating.

Now, it is time for you to take what you have learned and make it your own. Embrace the principles of calorie deficit cooking and let them guide you as you create your unique, personalized culinary masterpieces. Experiment, innovate, and explore new horizons. Allow your taste buds to be your compass, leading you towards combinations that delight and energize you.

Remember that your feedback is invaluable. As you embark on your own calorie deficit journey, I encourage you to share your experiences, discoveries, and adaptations of the recipes in this book. Your insights will not only inspire others but also contribute to the collective knowledge and evolution of calorie deficit cooking.

Share your stories, your successes, and even your challenges. Together, we can build a supportive community that uplifts and motivates one another on this path towards a healthier, happier life. Your voice matters, and your feedback will shape future editions of the Calorie Deficit Cookbook, ensuring its relevance and effectiveness for generations to come.

I am honored to have been a part of your transformation, and I am confident that the principles and recipes you have encountered in this book will continue to serve you well. But above all, I want you to remember that this journey is about more than just weight loss. It is about reclaiming your power, nurturing your body, and cultivating a positive relationship with food.

As you close this book, may you carry the lessons you have learned and the flavors you have savored in your heart. Approach each meal with intention, gratitude, and a sense of adventure. Let every bite be a celebration of the incredible person you are and the remarkable journey you are on.

Thank you for embarking on this remarkable adventure with me. Your dedication to your well-being inspires me, and I am grateful to have had the opportunity to be a part of your transformation. As you step forward into the world, remember that you are capable of achieving anything you set your mind to. Embrace the power of calorie deficit cooking, and let it propel you towards a future filled with health, vitality, and joy.

Wishing you a life brimming with flavor, wellness, and boundless possibilities.

30-DAY CALORIE DEFICIT TRACKER

DAY	DATE	DAILY CALORIE INTAKE	CALORIES BURNED	CALORIE DEFICIT	WEIGHT CHANGE
1					
2					
3					
4					
5					
6					
7					
8					
9					
10					
11					
12					
13					
14					

15					
16					
17					
18					
19					
20					
21					
22					
23					
24					
25					
26					
27					
28					
29					
30					

Printed in Great Britain
by Amazon

42106084R00040